HEALING GIFTS

Qi Gong
in Breast Cancer Recovery

Margaret Randolph & Cielle Tewksbury

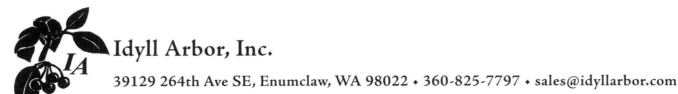

Idyll Arbor, Inc.

39129 264th Ave SE, Enumclaw, WA 98022 ✦ 360-825-7797 ✦ sales@idyllarbor.com

Library of Congress Cataloging-in-Publication Data

Randolph, Margaret, 1948-
 Healing gifts : qi gong in breast cancer recovery / Margaret Randolph & Cielle Tewksbury.
   p. cm.
 Includes bibliographical references.
 ISBN 978-1-882883-75-2 (alk. paper)
 1. Breast--Cancer--Patients--Rehabilitation. 2. Qi gong. I. Tewksbury, Cielle, 1938- II. Title.
 RC280.B8R36 2009
 362.196'994490092--dc22
 [B]
                              2009013747

ISBN 9781882883752

The information in this book is offered as a complement, not as a substitute for prescribed medical treatment. It is essential that the reader be in consultation with her physician during the course of recovery.

Contents

Gratitudes

A community of friends have given support, advice, and encouragement during the creation of this book. We would especially like to thank Chungliang Huang, Tai Ji master and founder of Living Tao Foundation, who has widened our horizons and given us courage to create. Heart-felt thanks to Lucy Hohn, who volunteered to be our "production team." This never would have happened without her. Thanks for the patience and skills of Yada Claassen and William F. Hull, who helped us through the photographic experience. Thanks to Leslie Richardson and Mary Brown Sinclair for their thoughtful editing. And, thanks to our many Tai Ji friends near and far.

Introduction

Sometimes healing

Needs no words

But happens

One small moment

At a time

Around the edges

Like stars

On a spring night

Each one

Bringing its small gift

Of light

And hope

Enough to bear

Us home

Across the twilight.

—Lois Bresee

A Word From Cielle Tewksbury

The word "recovery," according to Webster's dictionary, comes from the Latin word "recipere" to receive; to assimilate through the mind and senses; to restore to usefulness.

Each one of us, in our journey back, will discover many roads to our recovery. In this manual, we offer you one pathway that is drawn from the Chinese practice of Qi Gong. This gentle approach is like standing quietly with open hands and heart, listening, allowing, and accepting the possibility of healing. There are hundreds of rehabilitation programs available to those in recovery. They all have excellent merits. In this approach, we hope to address more than just the physical aspects of healing. We will combine the physical principles and enhance them with the use of visual images.

These positive emotional and mental pictures strengthen and encourage the body toward healing. Such a gentle and nurturing approach blends the body, mind, and spirit, and guides us on this receptive path to recovery.

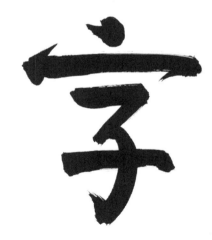

A Word From Meg. Randolph

The practice of Qi Gong opens the body's energy channels to healing. Where no disease exists, it is preventive medicine, keeping the channels open to prevent injury, illness, or emotional imbalance. When disease is present and the energy channels are blocked, Qi Gong facilitates the opening of the channels and the promotion of healing. Since Qi Gong addresses the emotional, physical, and spiritual aspects of healing, it is of the utmost benefit for those healing from disease.

As a physical therapist, I have spent years teaching women who have had mastectomies a series of range of motion and stretching exercises to increase movement and function. While this was beneficial, I felt there was something missing. I did not find that my clients were particularly engaged in the exercises; rather they found the exercises to be painful and boring. One day, as a client was leaving the office, it occurred to me that many of the movements I do in my Tai Ji and Qi Gong practice would help attain the physical therapy goals of increasing range of motion and function. I also realized Qi Gong would afford a better sense of well-being and relaxation since the movements address all aspects of healing. I asked my client to stay a while longer and I gave her some simple Qi Gong movements. Gradually, as she practiced the movements, I saw a face of stone soften and become relaxed. Not only did this woman reach a greater range of motion, she had a much more positive attitude about her body. The movement was focused on what worked and felt good, rather than on what was painful and difficult. The coordinated breathing promoted relaxation and increased range of motion. From that day forth I have used my Qi Gong practice to work with people who have limited upper extremity mobility.

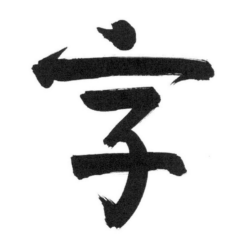

Anecdote From Sally Peavy

A diagnosis of breast cancer takes your breath away when first heard. It comes about after doctor appointments, tests, biopsies, and literally stops you in your tracks. It is unfortunately a common denominator for many women, and many women have gone ahead of us in this battle. Today there are many options for women facing this diagnosis, and the prognosis is very good for most women. The time after the diagnosis and during various treatments should be spent in ways that help one feel whole, positive, and nurtured.

For many years I noticed in TV programs, films, and articles, that there was a healing art called Tai Ji that had been practiced for thousands of years in China. It seemed to me to combine a sense of stillness with movement and meditation. As I learned more about it, I became even more intrigued. I began taking Tai Ji and Qi Gong classes two years before my diagnosis of breast cancer and was instantly struck with how spiritual and meditative the movements were. They brought about an inner calm and sense of connectedness to the earth. Yes, there were many things to remember when learning Tai Ji and Qi Gong, as there are with any new practices. However, very soon the movements themselves, whether done to music or outside as a part of nature, take over and seem to bring about an awareness of ordinary life that had not been present before. I began to develop a feeling of oneness with life that I had not previously taken time to find. The breathing and ritual movements calmed my inner tensions and turbulent thoughts, even going so far as to help relax my perpetually tense shoulder muscles.

There are many life-altering events that we face during our time on this earth. We are constantly bombarded by noise, chaos, and a whirlwind of new information every day. For me, practicing Qi Gong has helped quiet the turbulent storm of daily living, helped settle my thoughts concerning my personal battle with breast cancer, and provided peace and stillness, all the while creating a sense of awareness and connectedness that is very spiritual in nature. I wish for you these same blessings.

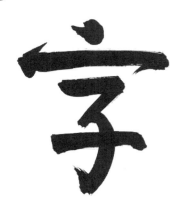

Anecdote From Meredith Morgan

After a mastectomy in 1996, I could not move my left arm, was quite weak, and could only sustain movement for five to ten minutes. A friend suggested that I try Qi Gong and I began private lessons in my home. Gradually I was able to increase my range of motion, improve my breathing, and strengthen my whole body. I not only felt better physically, but also emotionally and mentally. The use of images and the gentle flow of the movements was such a gift to the healing process. It gave me hope and a confidence that I could improve and be in charge of my life again. Studying Qi Gong and Tai Ji has become a major part of my life and given me a new world to explore and share with others.

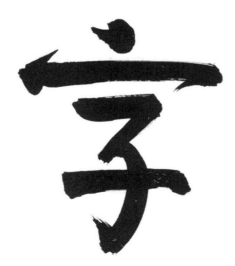

Essentials

Qi Gong

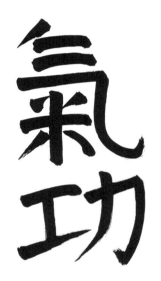

Qi Gong comes from the Chinese words "Qi" meaning "energy" or "life force," plus "Gong," which translates as "work" or "practice." As a complementary form of medicine, it is highly effective for those recovering from illness. Qi Gong, along with Tai Ji and acupuncture, have been practiced in China for over two thousand years.

This ancient form of Chinese healing has often been called a moving meditation because the practice works with body, mind, and spirit to restore balance, revitalize energy, and calm the mind. It uses a variety of images from animal life and the natural world around us to focus the mind. This, along with correct posture and deep breathing, helps to bring us to a state of relaxed, quiet awareness.

Unlike most exercises offered in recovery, Qi Gong places the emphasis on the ability of the mind to affect the body through the use of imagination and visualization. This focused concentration sends a positive message to the body that encourages the healing process. The movements are gentle and slow, requiring minimal physical effort, thus making them ideal for those experiencing cancer-related fatigue.

Exercise

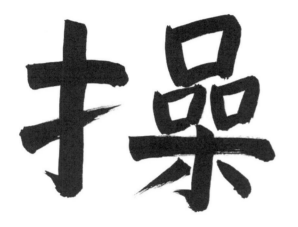

During recovery, it is essential to overcome fatigue. Current literature on cancer recovery recommends exercise such as walking programs and aerobics. When challenged by cancer-related fatigue, thoughts of strenuous exercise may be overwhelming. Qi Gong movement, although slow and gentle, offers the same benefits as a more strenuous exercise program.

Movement increases energy and boosts the immune system. Some of the side effects of chemotherapy, such as neutropenia (low white blood count) and thrombocytopenia (low platelet count), can be diminished through exercise. A normal white blood count is a defense mechanism against disease. A normal platelet count prevents bruising and bleeding. Certain Qi Gong movements are designed to boost the immune system. By providing deep relaxation, Qi Gong promotes emotional balance. Through the practice, a deep sense of well-being is felt. All of these factors combine to increase function and improve quality of life.

Wu Wei

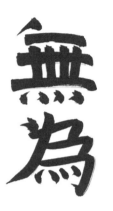

There are two Chinese characters which exemplify our ability to listen to and balance the changing needs of our body. Wu Wei asks us to accept the give and take that life demands of us, to be able to let things come to us with the same ease we let things go. It is like water that chooses to move around an obstacle rather than struggling to go through it: the essence of "going with the flow."

Balance

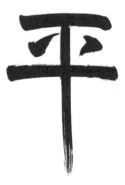

A sense of balance is a fundamental concept in Qi Gong. On a physical level, we are learning to pay close attention to the messages the body gives and to adjust or modify our practice accordingly. Many times, how we feel emotionally influences our daily practice. Learning to find a balance between what our body tells us and how we are feeling emotionally is an important tool in the process of recovery. Gently accepting the changing flow we experience helps us to respect the individual way our body is healing.

Listening to Our Bodies

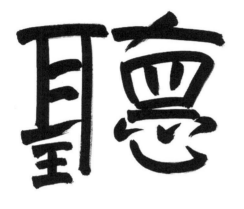

Listening to our bodies is an important key to all exercise. When we experience fatigue, it is sometimes difficult to push ourselves to move. On the other hand, pushing too hard can be harmful. One of the lessons of Qi Gong is balance—both physical and emotional. To find this balance, it is important to learn how to modify the movements.

There are several ways to do this:

- Decrease the size of a movement if it is uncomfortable or tiring. For example, if it is painful or tiring to raise the arm above shoulder height, keep the movement lower.

- Vary the repetitions of a movement. For instance, begin with three repetitions, increase to five, seven, etc.

- Vary the frequency of the exercise. Instead of five times a week, try three times a week.

- Vary the duration of the exercise. Begin with five or ten minutes of exercise and gradually increase.

Heeding the Precautions

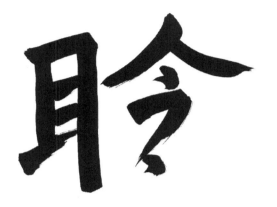

First and foremost, one must follow the recommendations of the physician. This is particularly important for women who have undergone reconstructions, such as TRAM or latissimus flaps, or who are undergoing chemotherapy. One must be mindful of swelling or lymphedema. Over-exercising can increase edema; however, it is important to continue with modified movements. Finding balance between rest and exercise is essential to the practice. More information on this is available in the section that follows on lymphedema.

There are various other side effects of chemotherapy, depending on the type. It is recommended that before beginning any exercise program, you discuss it with your health care provider.

When the platelets are low, precaution is advised for massage, acupuncture, or acupressure since bruising or bleeding could occur. This should be based on your lab values and cleared with your physician.

When there is fibrosis from radiation, care must be used with stretching exercises. The movements must be slow, gentle, and with a prolonged stretch. Never force the movement.

Good hand washing cannot be emphasized enough, both for you and the people with whom you come in contact. This is the first and simplest line of defense against disease and is particularly important when the immune system is compromised.

Times when exercise needs to be minimal to none.

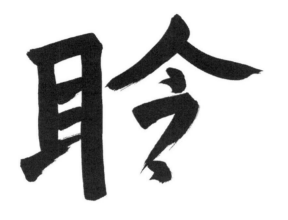

Acute Infection	No Exercise
Hemoglobin	
Less than 8 g/dl	No Exercise
8-10 g/dl	Light Exercise
White Blood Count	
Less than 500/mm³	No Exercise
Greater than 500/mm³	Light Exercise
Platelet Count	
Less than 5,000 mm³	No Exercise
5,000 - 50,000/mm³	Light Exercise
Bone Metastasis	
Involves more than 50% of bone cortex	No Exercise
Involves 25-30% of bone cortex	Partial weight bearing and light exercise with no stretching

In cases where there are cardiac conditions, such as cardiomyopathy, related to chemotherapy or radiation, your doctor should be consulted before beginning an exercise program.

(from workshop manual, "Treatment of Cancer Related Fatigue," Sharon Konecne, MHS, PT, 2005)

Edema Prevention and Reduction

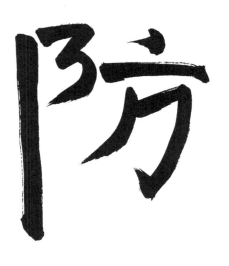

When lymphedema is present in the arms and hands, it is important to exercise; however, exercise must be done with caution. An increase in swelling indicates the exercise is too strenuous, so begin gently, slowly, and with frequent rest breaks. Gradually add exercise as you are able. Contracting and relaxing the muscles creates a pumping motion that helps move fluid out of the extremity. Deep breathing helps increase the flow of lymph fluid.

In the presence of lymphedema, it is recommended initially to consult a lymphedema specialist, such as an Occupational or Physical Therapist with specialized training in creating exercise programs for lymphedema. It is usually recommended that the exercise be done with a custom-made compression garment on the involved arm. Your physician or therapist will be able to refer you for a fitting.

To prevent complications from lymphedema, take care to avoid cuts, scratches, and irritations. If you sew, protect your fingers by using a thimble. Keep hands moisturized to prevent dryness and cracking.

Wear gloves for dish washing and yard work. Wash cuts and cover immediately. Use care when shaving underarms. No injections, blood draws, or blood pressures should be taken on the involved arm.

Carrying a heavy purse is not good for your back or your operative side. Pressure on your involved arm from a purse or a tight bra strap can cause swelling. Scale down; carry a small purse and carry it on the uninvolved side. Tight clothing or jewelry should be avoided on the involved arm. Take care around hot objects, wear sunscreen when you are outdoors, and use insect repellent to prevent bites and stings.

Alignment

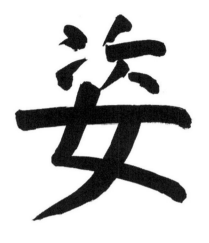

Good posture or alignment is never fixed or rigid, but comes from the elasticity, responsiveness, and adaptability of our bones, muscles, and tendons.

If we think of the body as composed of separate masses: head, chest, and pelvis, our body becomes most stable and aligned when the center of gravity of each of these masses can be lined up over each other. Rhythmical, even breathing coupled with relaxed muscles can allow the body to find its natural alignment. Holding the breath or tightening the muscles limits our ability to find our center and almost always pulls us off balance.

Developing the ability to sense the body in space as a three dimensional object can be a great aid to posture.

Most of us are aware of the front of the body; it takes practice to sense the sides and back as well.

Following are some suggestions for sensing your alignment:

- Standing quietly, become aware of your breathing and feel the weight of your bones and muscles. Shift the weight forward, backward, and around on your feet and notice how the rest of your body responds in an effort to maintain balance.

- Jut your chin forward and then pull it backward and again feel how your body adjusts.

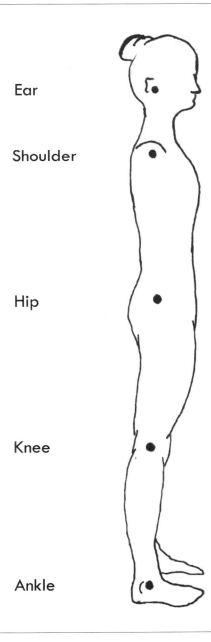

Ear

Shoulder

Hip

Knee

Ankle

- Imagine the center of your feet extending down beneath the earth and your head expanding up toward the sky. Feel the breath and the flow of energy traveling easily up and down the length of your body.

- Sense a line traveling down the front of your body from the tip of the nose, the sternum, the belly button, and the pubis. Gently tap each of these locations.

- Draw another line from your earlobes, tip of your shoulder, side of the hips, side of the knees, and the ankle bone.

- Draw a third line from the back of your head, between the shoulder blades, down through the sacrum and out the coccyx, like a tail, extending down to the earth.

Touch the crown of your head. Imagine a weighted line dropping straight down through the center of your head, center of the torso, and center of the pelvis. Think of the pelvis as a bowl of water with the dan tien (energetic center below the navel in the belly) floating in the center of your body.

This stretching up of the head to heaven and of the tail bone down to earth creates space in the body's trunk, allowing the organs to work more efficiently.

Breath

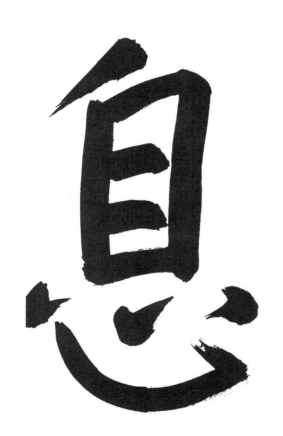

Breathing in,

I am a mountain,

imperturbable,

still,

alive,

vigorous.

Breathing out,

I feel solid.

The waves of emotion

can never carry me away.

from Breathing, **Call Me By My True Names***, Thich Nhat Hanh*

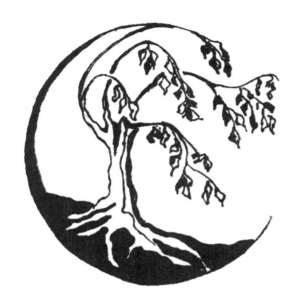

Like the sap rising and falling within a tree, the breath is the nourishment that feeds the heartwood of the body, rooting us in the earth, flowing through us and lifting us to the sky.

The way we breathe and the way we stand are interdependent. Any change in our posture will affect the breathing process; any change in the way we breathe will affect our alignment. The diaphragm is the most important muscle for breathing. It functions as the base of support for the heart and lungs as well as the roof for the organs of the abdominal cavity. It is the great connector between the heart and the body itself since two of its tendons, called cruras, connect upward to the pericardium, which holds the heart, and downward to the first, second, and third lumbar vertebrae.

All Qi Gong exercises incorporate attention to the breath. The lift and fall of the movement is mirrored by the lift and fall of the breath as if the movement itself were floating on the breath. The simple act of focusing upon the breath, listening to what our body needs, almost always will slow and deepen the act of inhalation and exhalation. There are no set rules for breathing. In general, raising movements are done on an inhalation, whereas sinking or lowering movements happen on the exhalation.

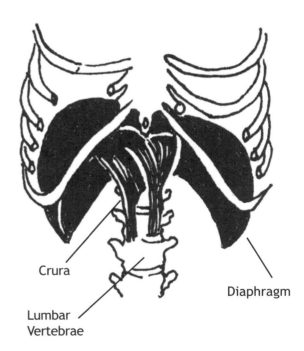

Crura

Lumbar
Vertebrae

Diaphragm

Breathing Practices

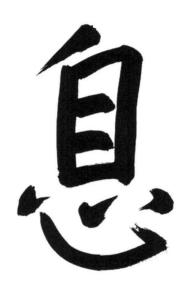

All of the breathing practices can be done either standing, sitting, or lying down.

Before each Qi Gong Practice, take a moment to listen to your breathing. Allow the breath to slow and deepen. Gently let the incoming breath expand down and out to the sides, as if an umbrella were slowly opening inside you. This is called belly or abdominal breathing and is what you see in the breathing patterns of babies. Be aware of the breath expanding the rib cage to the front, side, and back. Imagine the breath descending all the way down to your toes as you inhale, and rising all the way out the top of your head as you exhale.

Dan Tien Breathing

	吸	呼
Lower Dan Tien	Begin with your hands on the belly. **INHALE,** expand hands out from the belly.	**EXHALE,** bring hands in to the heart.
Middle Dan Tien	**INHALE,** expand hands away from heart.	**EXHALE,** bring hands to the forehead, gently covering eyes with hands.
Upper Dan Tien	**INHALE,** expand hands away from forehead.	**EXHALE,** lower hands to sides of the body.

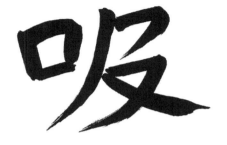

Embrace the Circle

- Beginning with your hands at your sides, *INHALE*, lift hands, palms up, through the center of the body above the head.

- Raise the arms to your own comfort level. *EXHALE*, separate hands to the sides and draw a circle around the body.

Embrace Tiger, Return to Mountain

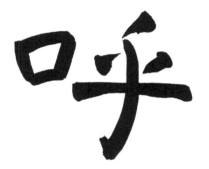

- *INHALE*, cross hands at wrists, palms facing you, hands at heart level.

- *EXHALE*, turn palms down and float hands downward.

Lotus Opening & Closing

- Imagine a lotus blossom between your hands, held at the level of your belly (dan tien).

- Breathe in and let the hands expand, as if the blossom were opening.

- Breathe out and let the blossom close, still leaving some space between the hands.

This is a relaxing breath that also creates energy in the palms of your hands.

Qi Gong Movement

The Qi Gong movements are divided into four levels, moving through the various stages of recovery.

1. *Early, Gentle Motion*—Level one addresses movements for the days immediately following surgery. During these early days after surgery the movements focus only on fingers, elbows, and shoulders. These exercises promote circulation into the area and help decrease pain and swelling. They can be done while lying down or sitting.

2. *Beginning to Move*—Level two offers suggestions for movements which are below shoulder height. These exercises begin to increase the joint mobility and help prevent tissue tightening.

3. *Starting to Reach*—When the arms are able to move above shoulder height, level three offers Qi Gong movements which further restore mobility and increase function.

4. *Reaching for Full Function*—The fourth level provides movements appropriate when you can reach fully above your head. They restore full mobility and function in the shoulder and arm.

Remember:

- Although the movements are shown in a standing position, they can be adapted for sitting, and some can be practiced while lying down.

- When doing the Qi Gong in a standing position, the knees are never locked, but slightly bent.

- It is of the utmost importance that you do each exercise to your own comfort level.

- The goal is to gain your normal mobility in the shoulder and chest, but not at the cost of increasing pain or swelling.

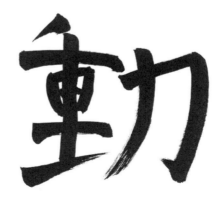

Early Gentle Motion

Fingers & Wrists

These are usually appropriate from one day post-op through week one.

Finger and wrist exercises can be done seated or standing.

1 Lift your arms in front of you, palms up.

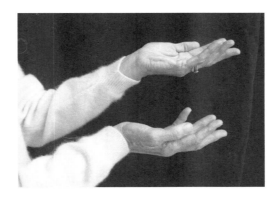

2 Curl fingers into palms, beginning with the little finger.

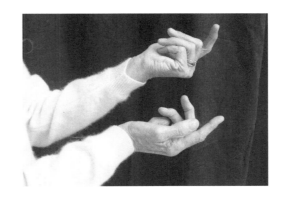

3 Place thumb over the fingers.

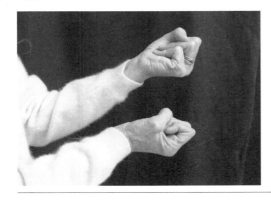

4 Rotate the wrists.

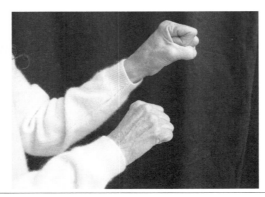

5 Extend fingers out straight, then relax hands and lower arms.

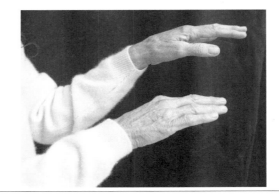

Repeat steps 1–5, moving arms out to side.

Elbows

- Lying on your back or sitting, begin with your arms at your sides.

- Bend your elbow, allowing your palm to face your chest, and gently walk your fingers across your chest to your opposite shoulder.

- From that position, straighten your elbow and let your forearm return to the starting position

- Do on both sides.

Shoulder Rolls

- Sitting or standing in erect posture, slowly roll your shoulders backwards several times, then forwards several times.

- The emphasis should be on moving your shoulder blades back towards each other with the tips pointing downward.

Shoulder Blade Squeezes

- Sitting or standing in erect posture, with the tips of the shoulder blades pointed downward, squeeze the shoulder blades towards each other.

- You should feel a stretch across your chest as you do this. This is a good stretch for the chest muscles.

- Hold this for 5–15 seconds, to your own comfort level.

Beginning to Move

Water Beads on Lotus Leaf

1 Begin with hands at dan tien level (slightly below the navel), left hand above the right, palms facing each other with space in between.

Slowly circle left hand clockwise, then counterclockwise, feeling the energy within the space between your hands.

Rotate your hands, bringing the right hand above the left and circle it both directions also.

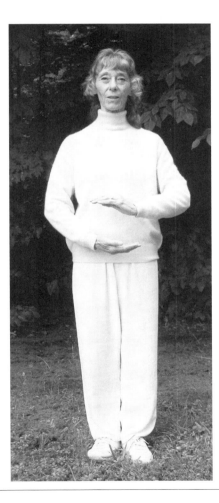

2 Then open your palms outward, as if pouring the water beads to the earth.

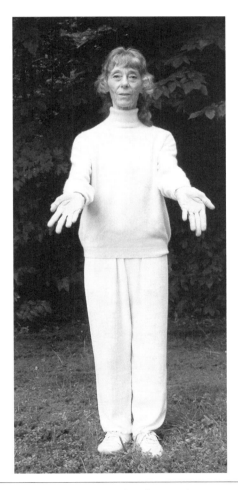

Spring Silkworm Gathering Silk

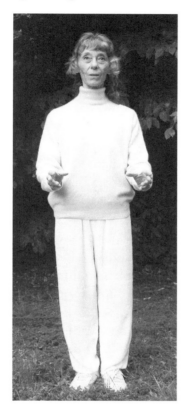

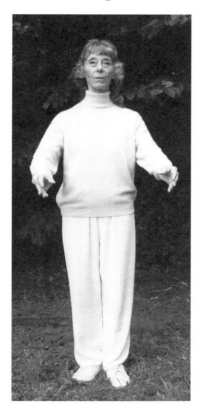

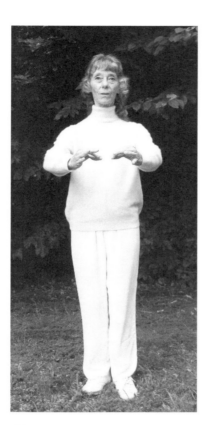

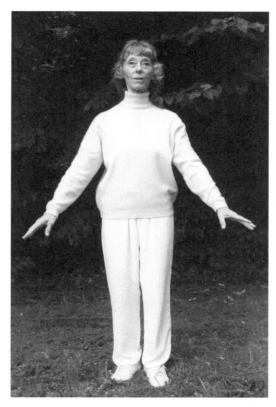

1 INHALE, bending the elbows, slowly raise wrists to waist height.

2 EXHALE, extend elbows at heart level, fingers relaxed in front of you.

3 INHALE, join thumb and first finger of each hand, as if holding a silk cocoon.

Slowly draw hands out to the sides, as if drawing a silk thread from a cocoon.

4 EXHALE, release the threads and slowly lower arms to your sides.

Pushing Away Negativity, Bringing in Goodness

1 Stand with left foot forward. Right foot is turned slightly outward.

Push arms forward with palms facing away from you. Imagine as you push forward that you are pushing away negativity.

Take care to keep the trunk upright; do not lean forward as you do this.

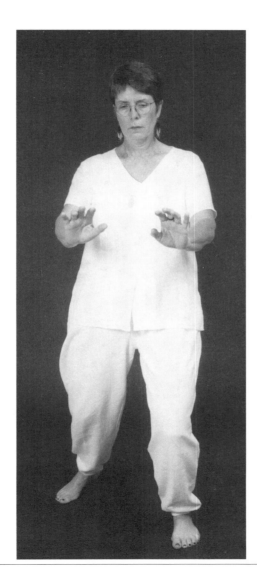

2 Pull arms in, palms facing toward you. As you pull in, you are pulling in goodness.

Repeat this with the right foot forward.

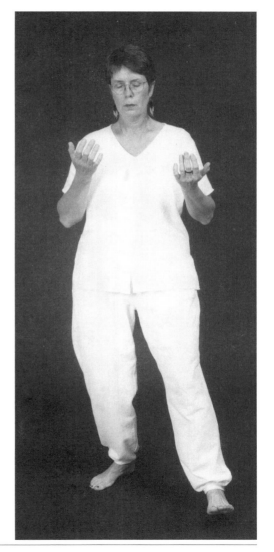

Gathering the Celestial Energies

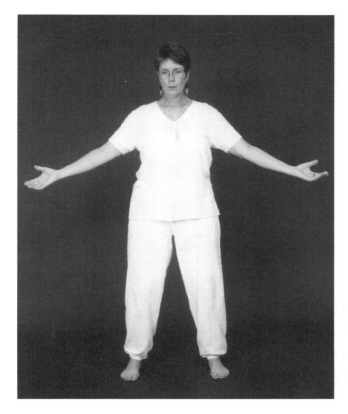 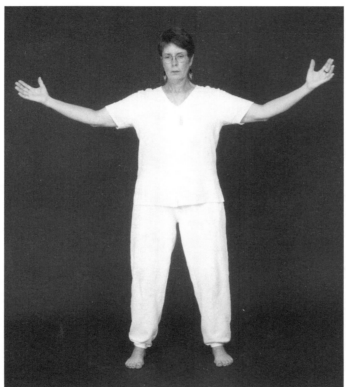 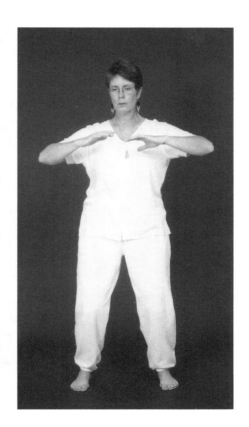

1 Begin with arms at sides, palms facing upwards, feet shoulder-width apart, knees gently bent.

2 Palms up, breathe in as arms lift out to sides, slightly below shoulder level. Increase height of the movement as tolerated.

3 Breathe out as arms fold inward, bending at elbows, palms down, gently pushing hands down to hip level while exhaling.

Balloon Inflating

1 Begin with feet shoulder-width apart, knees gently bent, arms relaxed at sides.

Breathe in as knees gently straighten and arms rise straight in front of you to slightly below shoulder level, palms down.

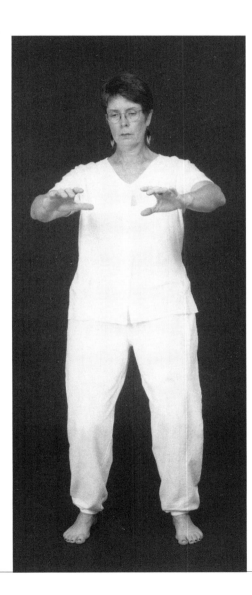

2 Breathe out slowly, bending knees gently, and pushing hands down to hip level.

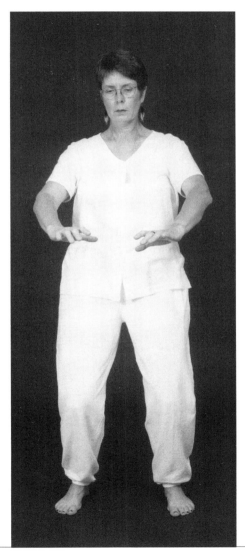

Illuminating the Mind: Dedicating the Heart and Mind to Peace and Healing

1 Begin with your feet shoulder-width apart, palms at your sides.

Move your palms to the sides of your head, but not touching your head.

Imagine that you are filling your palms with light and energy.

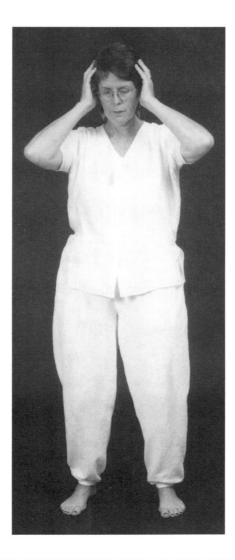

2 Move your hands away from the head, then back towards the head, but not touching the head.

Do this two times and then, on the third time, make circles with your hands.

Press hands down to hip level, reconnecting with the earth.

Imagine that you are filling your body with peace and healing.

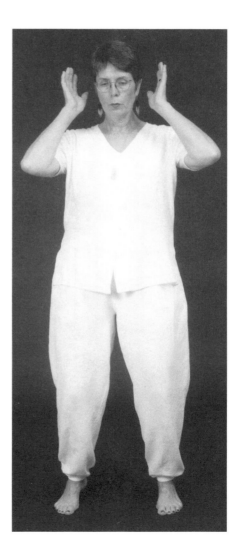

Starting to Reach

Fire and Water

1 Begin with weight on right foot and left foot forward, palms facing each other, shoulder-width apart, arms at hip level.

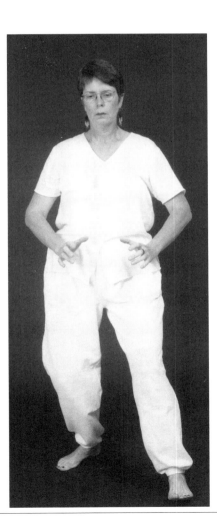

2 Shift weight onto left foot and draw a circle, moving forward and upward, over your head.

Shift weight back onto the right foot and lower hands back down to hip level.

Repeat this with your right foot forward.

This movement balances giving and receiving. It is a good time to reflect on all you have done for others and acknowledge that this may be your time to receive from others.

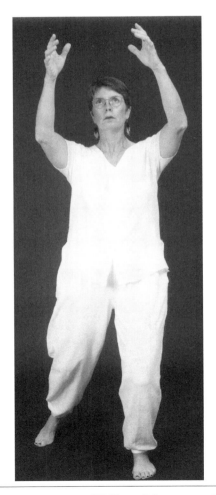

Wise Woman Listening

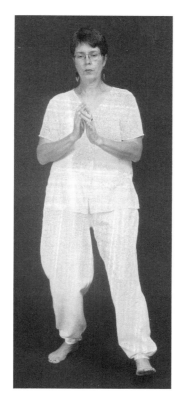

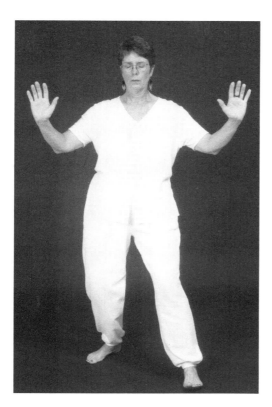

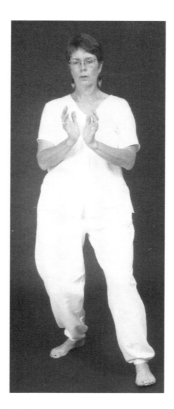

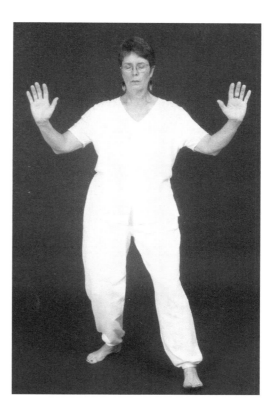

1 Begin with weight on right foot, left foot forward, knees gently bent, fingers loosely crossed over each other in prayer position.

2 Hands move slightly down, then spread apart to make a circle upward, closing back into prayer position.

As you do this, acknowledge your wisdom and ability to listen to your body.

3 As the prayer hands open like a flower, lift your arms upward from the heart to the crown of your head.

4 Offer your gifts of goodness, beauty, and wisdom. Circle your arms outward and back down to waist level.

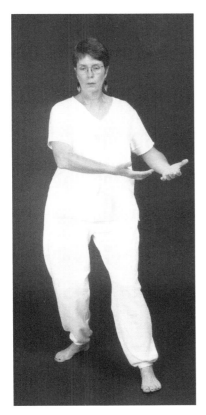

5 Palms face upward as you spread a circle clockwise three times.

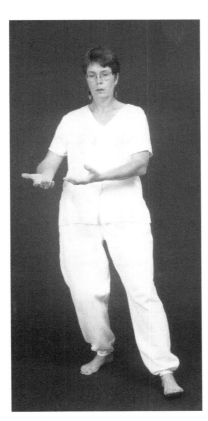

6 Receive the goodness and beauty of nature and the earth.

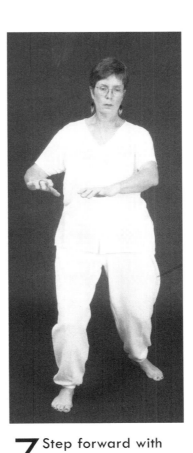

7 Step forward with your right foot.

Palms face downward as you spread a circle counterclockwise three times.

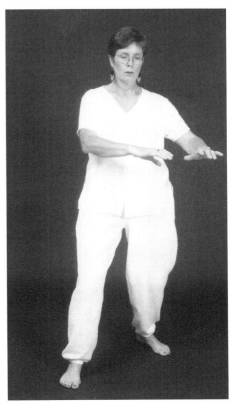

8 Send out light and energy as you reconnect to the earth.

Prayer Wheel

Hands rest on shoulders, elbows raised at sides to shoulder height, gently draw circles with the elbows.

Do three times forward and three times back.

To advance the movement, one elbow moves forward while the other moves backward.

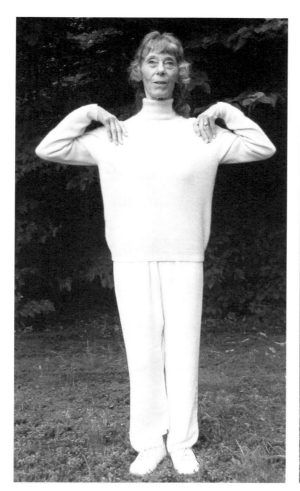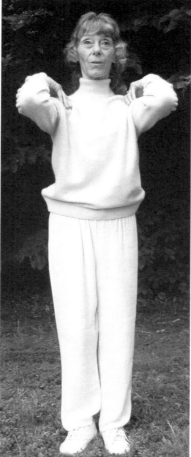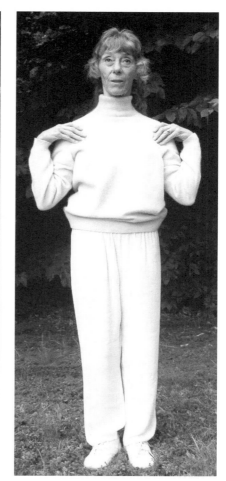

Dispelling Fear, Strengthening Courage

Place palms on your back at kidney level, fingers of each hand pointing slightly downward.

Gently circle the hands inward toward the spine and then outward toward the sides.

The emotions connected with the kidneys are fear and courage, so as you circle, you dispel fear and build courage.

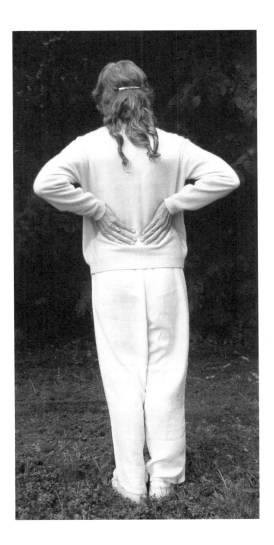

Clouds Passing

1 Stand with your feet shoulder-width apart.

Pull your right arm up through the center of your body, opening outward, as you shift your weight right.

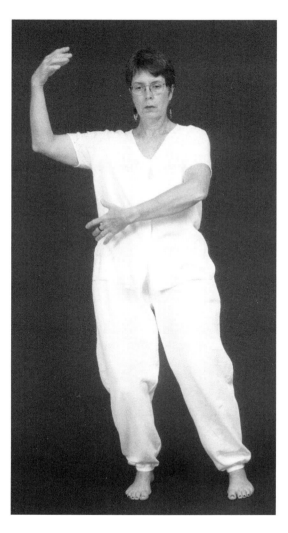

2 Repeat this move with your left arm, shifting your weight left.

Imagine that as you do this, whatever worries you may have will pass like the clouds.

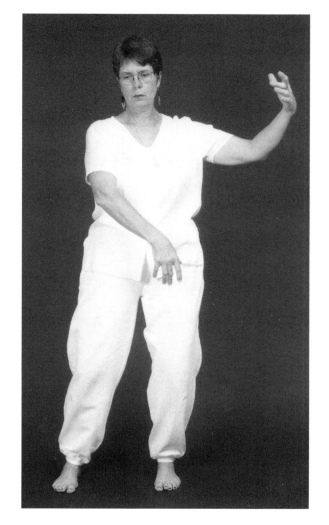

Reaching for Full Function

Opening the Sky Dome

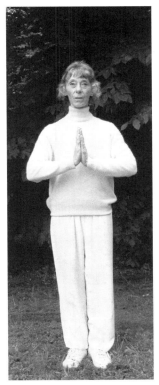

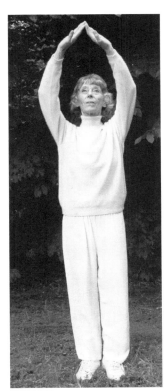

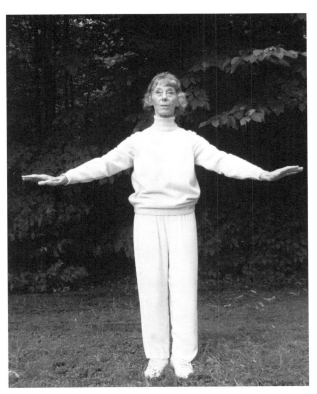

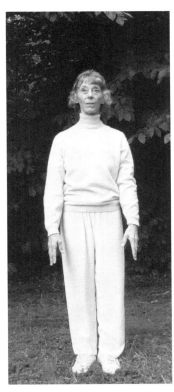

1 Stand with your feet together, hands in prayer position.

2 Lift hands up through center of your body.

Reverse hands so that they are touching back to back.

3 Press your hands open and lower to your sides.

4 End with hands at your sides.

Casting the Net, Reeling in the Stars

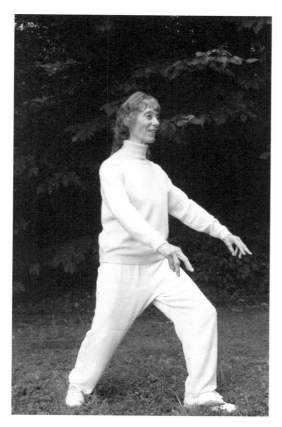

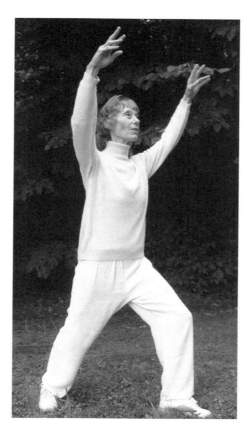

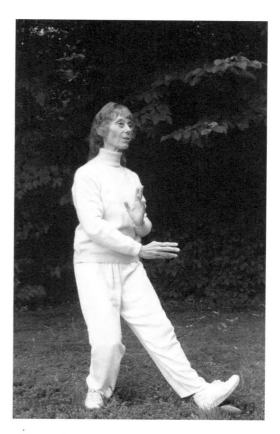

1 Start with feet at hip's width. Pivot left and step diagonally out with the left foot. Open arms out to sides.

2 Lift arms as if casting a net.

3 Shift weight back onto right foot, moving arms as if reeling in the net.

Repeat, pivoting and stepping diagonally with the right foot.

Picking the Peach

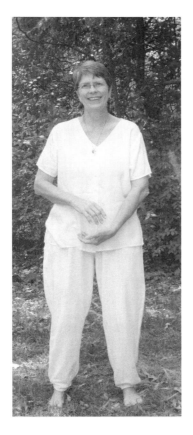 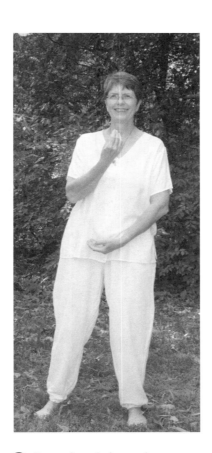 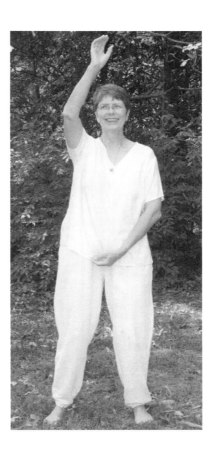 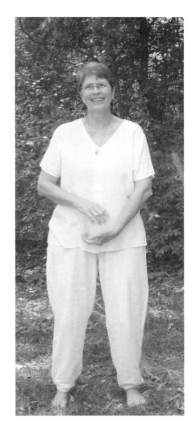

1 Begin with both hands resting in front of you at hip level.

Imagine the left hand is a basket, palm up, to receive the fruit.

2 Turn the right palm inward and begin to reach up as if you were picking a peach from a tree.

3 Turn the palm outward to pick the peach, then inward again.

4 Move the right hand downward to place the peach in the basket.

Repeat on the other side.

Balancing Energies

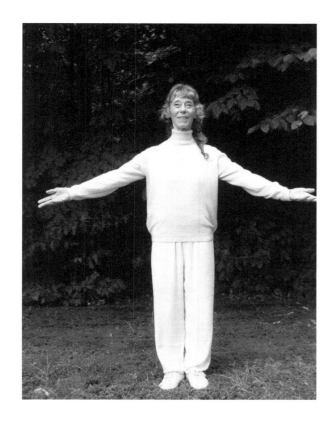

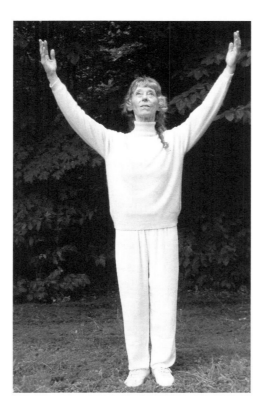

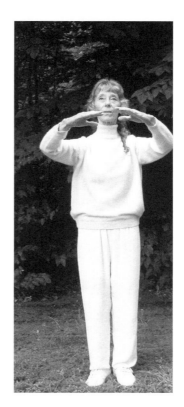

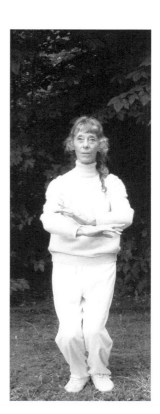

1 Gently lift arms out to your sides, slightly lower than shoulder height.

2 Lift arms overhead in a large circle, palms facing up to the sky.

3 Slowly lower both hands in front of you, palms down, until they reach waist level.

4 Bring your hands in to the center of your body, palms facing down.

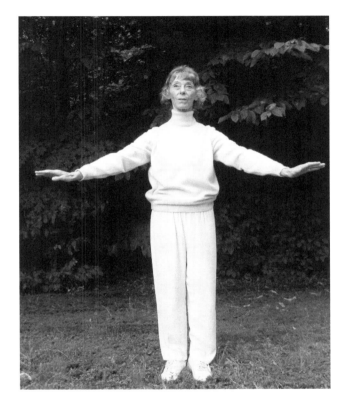

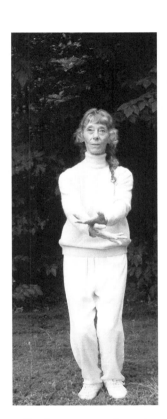

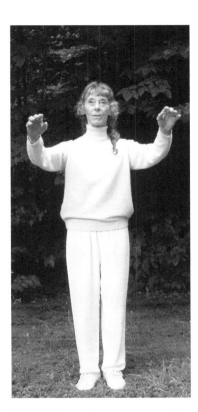

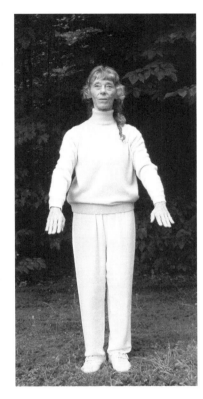

5 Move both hands in a circle, out and around to your sides, as if spreading over the earth.

6 Cross your hands at the wrist, palms up, as if lifting up the gifts from the earth.

7 Palms down, separate your hands and lower them down to your sides, returning the energy to the earth.

8 Once you lower your hands to your sides, swing the arms back out to your sides, and begin the entire sequence again.

White Crane Opens Her Wing

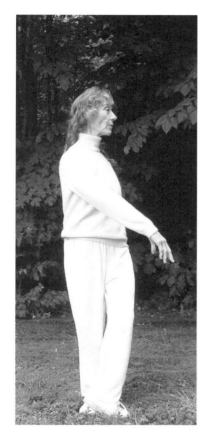 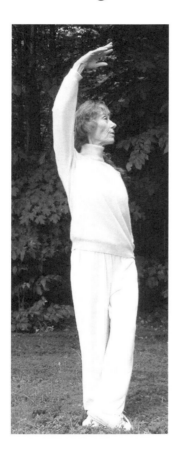 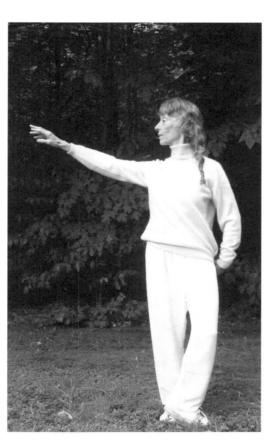 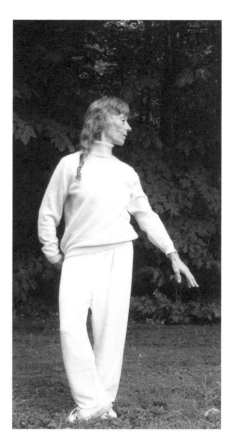

1 Stand, feet together. Inhale, bring left foot up to arch of right foot, turn upper torso to left as you circle right arm clockwise.

2 Rotate your torso right as you make the clockwise circle.

3 The left arm is like a wing resting at your side.

4 Repeat, stepping forward on the left foot with your right foot on the arch.

Illuminating the Crown: Receiving the Blessings of Life

1 Begin with your feet shoulder-width apart, palms at your sides.

Move your palms as if you were making a crown over your head.

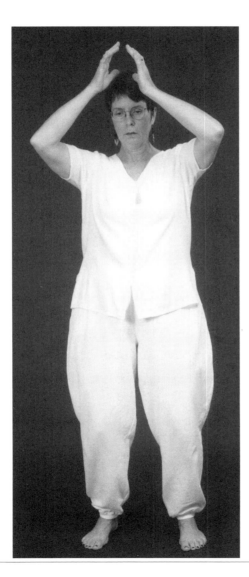

2 Open and close both hands two times. Repeat for a third time and this time make circles with your palms.

Press hands down to hip level.

Imagine that you are filling your body with peace and the blessings of life.

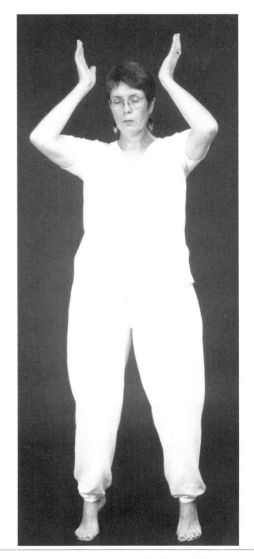

Useful Acupressure Points for Cancer Recovery

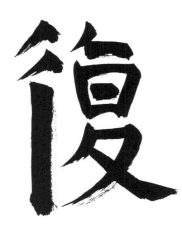

The practice of acupressure had its origins in China about 3,000 years ago. It is the foundation for the current practice of acupuncture, which uses needles to stimulate points along particular lines in the body. With acupressure the fingers are used to apply gentle pressure on the points.

A flow of energy follows particular lines throughout the body. These lines, called meridians, travel through the body and connect to the major organ systems. The lines are named for various organs in the body. However, the points may be used to treat symptoms unrelated to that specific organ.

By gently applying pressure to these points, the muscles surrounding the points relax, enabling blood and oxygen to flow to the affected area. Stimulating these points triggers the release of endorphins, which are substances in our bodies that when released, suppress pain. The Chinese call this "closing the pain gates." The relaxation of physical tension helps to calm the mind, and by reducing stress, we are aiding our recovery process.

These techniques can be useful in managing some of the various side effects of cancer treatment. Pain is often experienced during cancer recovery. There also may be side effects from chemotherapy. These vary depending on the therapy used. Some of the more common side effects are nausea and a compromised immune system. Here are a few simple acupressure techniques to help in cancer recovery.

When applying pressure to the points, use a thumb or finger. The nails must be cut short because the pressure is applied directly through the tip of the finger or thumb. The pressure is applied perpendicular to the point, not at an angle. Keep the finger joints relaxed. Apply pressure for up to one minute; less if symptoms resolve more quickly.

Pain

Large Intestine 4 – Hegu

This point is easily accessible for pain control. When pain is present, this point will feel extremely tender. Pressure on the point, while not comfortable initially, will eventually relieve pain. Hegu lies between the thumb and first finger in the web space where the 1st and 2nd metacarpal bones meet. This point is also useful for calming the mind.

This point should not be used during pregnancy as it may start labor contractions.

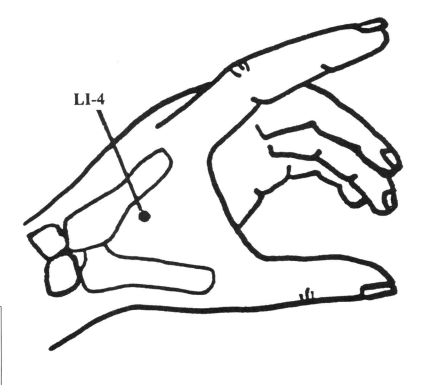

LI-4

Boosting the Immune System

Conception Vessel 17 – Dan Zhong

This point is in the center of the breast-bone, three thumb widths up from the tip of the breast bone. This point is also good for relieving anxiety. It is the place where the spirit and the heart reside.

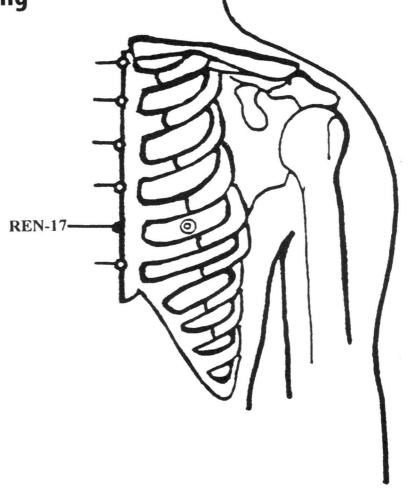

REN-17

Kidney 3 – Tai Xi

This point is on the inside of the foot between the ankle bone and the Achilles tendon, level with the top of the ankle bone.

It helps to calm the emotions, especially fear. It also brings qualities of stability, balance, and harmony.

It should not be used after the third month of pregnancy.

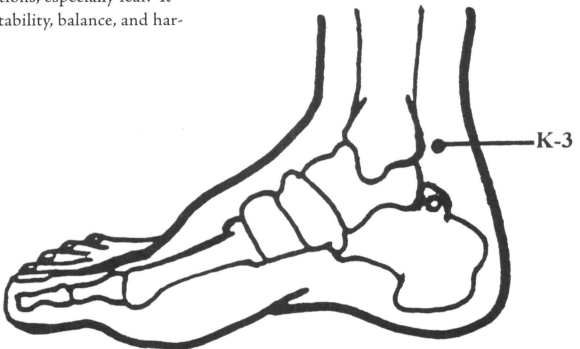

K-3

Liver 3 – Tai Chong

This point is in the valley between the big toe and the first toe.

It is useful for calming the spirit and easing depression, frustration, and anger.

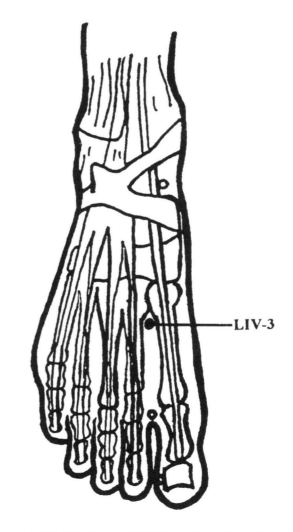

LIV-3

Lung 9 – Tai Yuan

This point is on the palm side of the forearm at the fold in the wrist on the thumb side of the arm. This is a strengthening and restorative point. It nourishes the spirit and opens the way to healing grief.

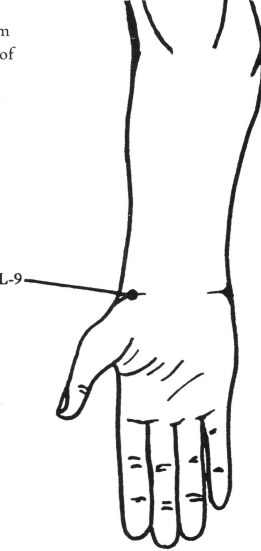

Large Intestine 11 – Qu Chi

This point is at the outer edge of the elbow crease when the elbow is bent to 90 degrees.

This is a very effective immune point. It is also a useful point for managing shoulder problems since it nourishes the muscles, joints, and tendons of the arm.

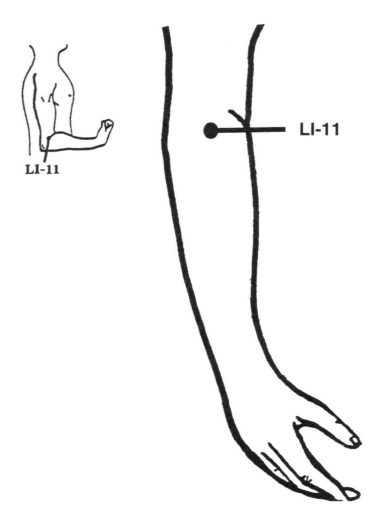

Nausea

Pericardium 6 – Nei Guan

This point is two thumb widths from the fold on the palm side of your wrist and between the two bones of your forearm. In addition to calming nausea and motion sickness, it protects the heart, both emotionally and physically, and promotes a sense of joy.

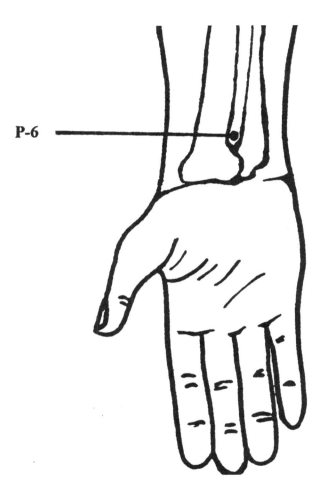

P-6

Quieting the Mind, Sleep Disturbance

Pericardium 8 – Lao Gong

Locate the point by bending your middle finger until it touches your palm. Once you have found the point, relax your middle finger. Use the opposite thumb or fingers to apply pressure to this point or make gentle circles over the point.

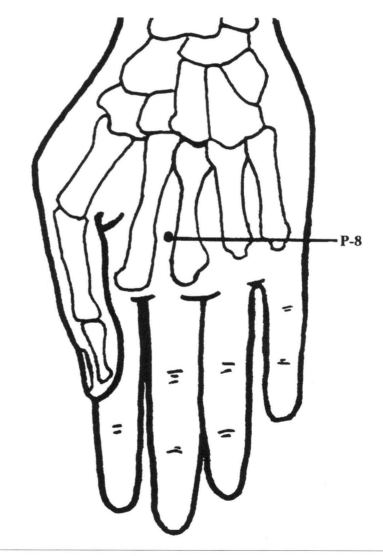

P-8

Relaxation

Finding balance between rest, relaxation, and movement is essential to recovery. Here we offer breathing techniques, self-massage, and meditation for relaxation.

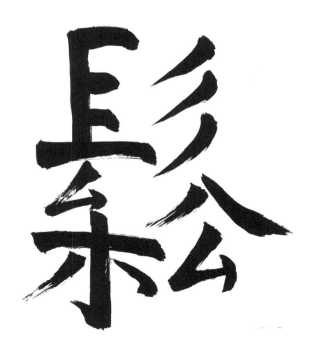

Circular Breath

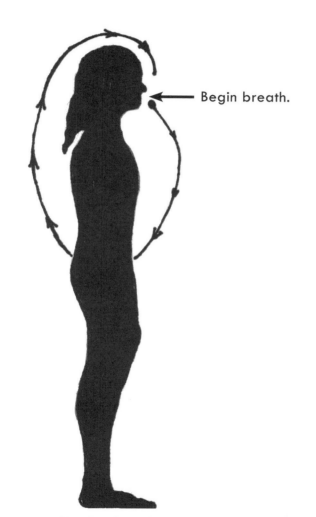

Begin breath.

Circular Breath

Deep breathing pumps the lymph fluid and may help decrease the effects of lymphedema.

Take a gentle breath in through your nose. Imagine this breath moving down the front of your body towards your lower abdomen, expanding the belly. The breath travels between your legs and, as you breathe out, imagine the breath moving up your spine, over your head and back through your nose.

Imagine yourself as a balloon filled with air – light and free.

Amazingly, we can forget to breathe, resulting in shallow breaths that do not fully nourish the body. It is a good practice to become conscious of your breathing. Find a way to incorporate conscious deep breaths into your daily routine. Perhaps remember to deep breathe at a stop light or when you're on the toilet. Breathing heals; it nourishes.

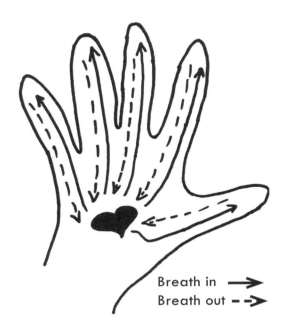

Breath in →
Breath out - ->

Start with little finger.
Left hand first.

Calming Breath

This is a simple breathing technique to decrease the stress of an existing or anticipated situation.

In the center of your palm there is an acupuncture point called Lao Gong. This point is a heart protector point. It is also called "the quieting the mind point." Focusing on the Lao Gong point is a good way to decrease stress and to help you sleep.

Start with your left hand. As you breathe in, take a finger of your right hand and trace a line from the Lao Gong point out to the tip of your small finger, trace the line back to Lao Gong, as you breathe out.

Continue until you have traced all five fingers of the left hand, then move to the right hand, beginning with the small finger. You can do this as many times as necessary to help you calm down or go to sleep.

Tapping the Windows of the Sky

This is a gentle and relaxing head massage. If you are uncomfortable reaching to your head, ask a friend to do this for you. Take both hands and gently use your fingers to tap your entire head, slowly moving your hands from one part of your head to another until your entire head has been gently tapped.

Releasing Negativity

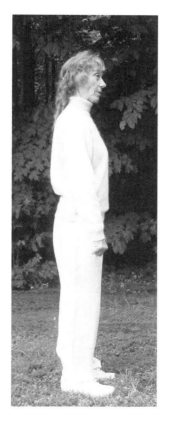 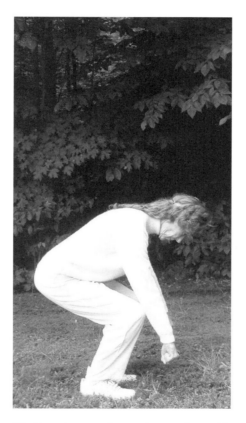 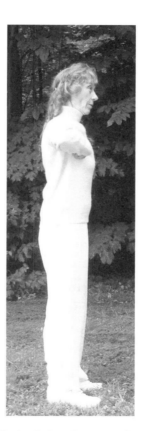 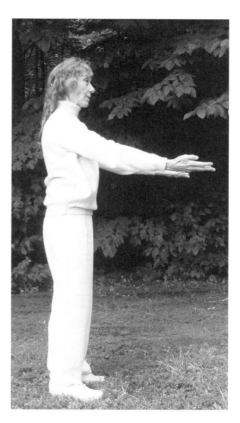

1 Begin in erect standing posture.

2 Bend over from the waist with knees bent.

Make fists with both your hands, as if holding whatever is negative.

3 Pull the fists up the sides of your body all the way to your armpits, as you come to stand.

4 Release the hands to the front while bending the knees slightly and expelling the breath.

Meditations

Spring Meditation

- Rest your hands on your knees, palms up.

- Turn palms to face earth, spread fingers like roots; lower hands towards the earth.

- Turn palms up, cup hands together as if holding a seed.

- Bring hands together, palms touching to form the shape of a bud.

- Lift hands to forehead and let the bud swell. Lift hands above the head, or to your comfort level, and open the fingers; the flower blooms.

- Separate the hands, slowly dropping the fingers downward as you lower the hands to let the petals fall.

- Turn the hands back to back, fingers pointing toward chest. Lift them in this position, up to the heart and rotate the wrists, pointing the fingers upward.

- Lift both hands to either side of your shoulders, palms facing behind you to signify the past, your ancestors, all that brought you to this present moment. Turn your palms to face forward and move them forward to the future.

- Bring the left hand under the right elbow as the upper torso turns to the right. Form a fist with the right hand for your strength.

- Open the fist slowly as you turn the torso to the left, and lower the right hand to the left elbow for your gentleness.

- Draw a circle with both hands and then return your hands to your knees.

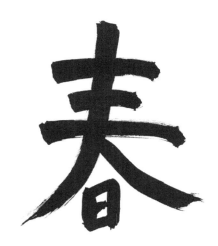

Compassionate Heart Meditation

- Seated, with feet shoulder-width apart and flat on the floor, close your eyes and connect to the earth through the balls of your feet.

- Imagine your feet have roots, connecting you to the earth.

- Focus your attention on your heart.

- As you breathe in, breathe the earth energy up your legs, into the abdomen, and then upward to fill your heart with earth energy.

- Breathe out, releasing any tensions and worries into the earth. Do this three times.

- Breathe in, continuing to fill yourself with energy – fire energy, creating a glow within you.

- Breathe out, imagining you are fanning a fire of light and healing.

- Breathe in, filling up with love, compassion, and healing for yourself.

- Breathe out, and continue to let go of your worries.

- Breathe in and fill with healing. Ask for what you need for yourself, remembering this is your time for yourself.

- Breathe out and as you are ready, open your eyes, remembering that each time you need to release tension and worry, you can find this quiet place within you that glows with love and nurturing for yourself.

Nurturing Yourself/Accepting Help

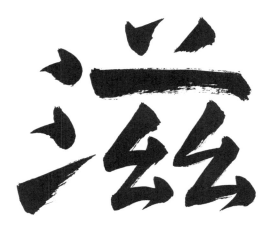

Qi Gong teaches balance between giving and receiving. Many of us spend a good portion of our lives giving. Learning to receive, to nurture ourselves, is often a difficult lesson. So, practice letting yourself accept help and practice nurturing yourself. Create quiet time for yourself, schedule massages, create time to write, read, listen to music, paint—whatever you love to do. Find time each day when you can focus on giving to yourself.

Practice saying "yes" to offers of help from others. Treasure your independence, but remember all the times you have reached out to help others.

Understand that this is your time to accept help. Accept it graciously, knowing this is an unconditional love offering from your friends and family.

Energy Conservation

During cancer recovery it is essential to practice energy conservation. It is important to balance exercise with rest and know how to pace yourself. Each day energy levels differ. Adjusting and adapting to the energy fluctuations is necessary.

Pacing can be accomplished by planning ahead, by looking at what you want to set out to do each day. Once you determine what you'd like to do, decide if it is realistic. Prioritize and delete activities as needed. Incorporate space and rest between activities. One of the lessons of Qi Gong is understanding the importance of space. This is an opportunity to learn about the importance of time and of creating space in your life.

Conserve energy by mixing low-energy-consuming tasks with higher-energy-consuming tasks. Learn how to decrease the energy needed for various tasks—sit on a stool at the kitchen sink to chop vegetables, use power tools to decrease consumption of your energy, sit on a tub chair for showering. Use good body mechanics when moving, but also when sitting to read, write, or use the computer. Poor posture consumes energy.

When doing household tasks, like vacuuming, use your legs to shift weight backwards and forwards, rather than leaning over the vacuum cleaner and pushing with the arms. Bend your legs while reaching down for an object on the floor, rather than bending your back. Maintain vertical trunk alignment as you do activities. Sit with the back well-supported, feet firmly planted on the floor, to allow you to receive earth energy. Keep the shoulder blades dropped and relaxed, chest stretched open, ears over the shoulders. Use a head set on your phone. Remember to breathe.

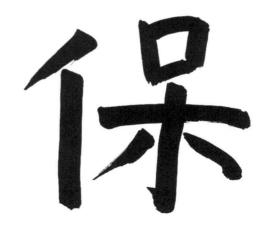

Sleep

Sleep gives the body an opportunity to heal and energy to replenish. Allow yourself at least eight hours of sleep at night. Nap during the day as needed. Use meditation techniques, breathing techniques, and acupressure points to promote relaxation. (Refer to the sections on breathing, meditation, and acupressure.)

Nutrition

Good nutrition is the key to healing, but good nutrition can be difficult when one is experiencing the side effects of chemotherapy, such as nausea and changes in sense of smell or taste. Stay well-hydrated and choose foods that provide good nutrition, as well as suit your tastes. If you are having difficulty eating, supplements may be needed. Consult a professional nutritionist who has experience with people who have cancer.

Positive Intention

Qi Gong clears the mind, helping one to feel grounded and connected. It offers a sense of well-being, clearing the mind, and unblocking areas of the body where energy is not flowing. It will open the doors to positive thinking, which helps promote healing. Negativity blocks energy flow and impedes the healing process. Keep an open heart and spirit as you move along the path of recovery.

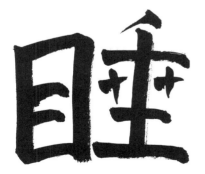

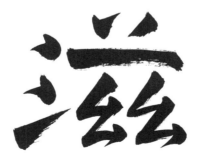

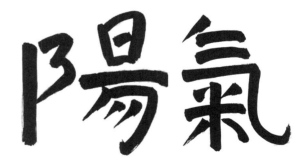

A Final Word

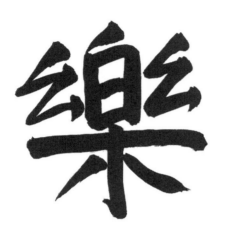

As we prepared **Healing Gifts**, we spent many moments of joy and laughter, practicing the breathing exercises, the movements, and editing the text. Although you may be experiencing some of the most challenging times of your life, we hope that you still may find moments of joyfulness and laughter. This too heals. Let your hands, feet, glands, and cells dance — and your souls awaken!

Laughter

What is laughter? What is laughter?

It is God waking up! O it is God waking up!

It is the sun poking its sweet head out

From behind a cloud

You have been carrying too long,

Veiling your eyes and heart

It is Light breaking ground for a great Structure

That is your Real body – called Truth

It is happiness applauding itself and then taking flight

To embrace everyone and everything in this world.

Laughter is the polestar

Held in the sky by our Beloved,

Who eternally says,

 "Yes, dear ones, come this way,

Come this way toward Me and Love!

Come with your tender mouths moving

And your beautiful tongues conducting songs

And with your movements – your magic movements

Of hands and feet and glands and cells – Dancing!

Know that to God's Eye,

All movement is a Wondrous Language,

And Music – such exquisite, wild Music!"

O what is laughter, Hafiz?

What is this precious love and laughter

Budding in our hearts?

It is the glorious sound

Of a soul waking up!

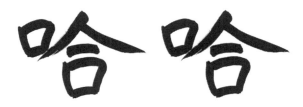

(*Laughter*, from ***I Heard God Laughing, Renderings of Hafiz***, Daniel Ladinsky)

Glossary of Chinese Calligraphy

Chinese is a symbolic, metaphoric language. We chose not to give "definitions" of the Chinese characters in the text with the hope that the reader could take a moment to reflect on the characters, letting them speak for themselves.

In this glossary of characters, you will find one or two possible English words for each character, however most characters have many possible and varied meanings. For some of the characters there will be further information about the characters within the main character. This opens the door to the symbolic nature of the language.

Following the glossary, there are six calligraphies, each with a poem by Cielle Tewksbury. The poems represent Cielle's metaphoric journey with the calligraphy. You may find that a particular calligraphy speaks to you and use this in your meditation or you might want to write your own poem or story.

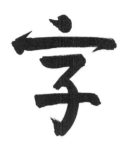

Zi - Word, character.
This character represents a child being born under a roof and symbolizes characters being created in the Chinese language.

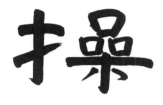

Cao - Exercise.
Hand, arm is the left hand character, symbolizing some type of action.

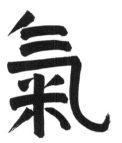

Qi (Chi) - Energy, vital life force.
The outside of this character is the symbol for vapor or steam. The inside character is rice. The steam cooks the rice, which gives us energy and sustains us.

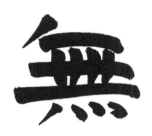

Wu - No, not.
This character is sometimes seen as a forest burning, leaving only seeds to sprout again from the earth.

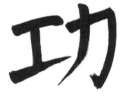

Gong - Strength, work.
The character on the left is work; the one on the right strength. Together they become skill.

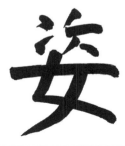

Zi - Posture, manner.
The bottom symbol is a woman.

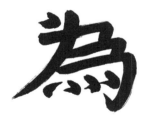

Wei - Do, doing.
This character is said to represent a hand leading an elephant. It can also be seen as power or potential energy. Wu and wei are used together to signify "not doing," letting things flow with nature.

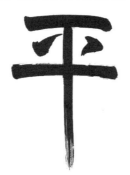

Ping - Balance, peace.
This character is like a balance scale. Through qi gong one finds emotional and physical balance.

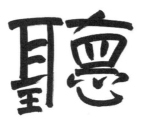

Ting - Listen, hear.
The top left hand character is an ear; the lower represents a king, queen, or ruler. The top right is mind; below it is an eye. The final two characters are one or oneness, and heart. All of these combined symbolize true, deep listening.

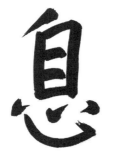

Xi - Breath.
The top character is self, natural; the bottom heart. To love oneself is to breathe. It is natural to breathe.

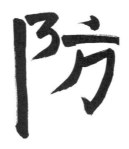

Fang - Prevent, guard against.
The left hand character represents a mound. The right hand character can mean direction or place. It can also signify a place of safety.

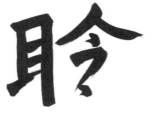

Ling - Listen, heed, pay attention to.
The left character is an ear. The right resembles a bell.

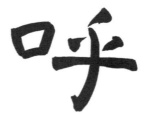

Hu - Exhale.
An open mouth on the left.

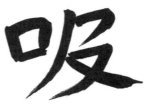

Xi - Inhale, suck.
An open mouth on the left.

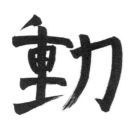

Dong - Motion, movement.
The right hand character means work.

Xin - Heart.
This character is a heart with its four chambers depicted.

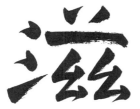

Zi - Nourish, nurture, support.
On the left is a symbol for water; on the right is silk.

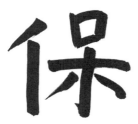

Bao - Protect, conserve.
An adult on the left, holding a baby on the right.

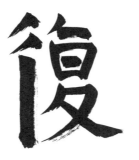

Fu - Recover, recovery, return.
Originally the upper right part represented a village and the lower a foot, thus someone returning. The square character can also represent the sun or the path of the sun returning.

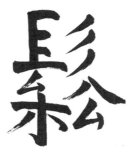

Song - Loose, relaxing.
This character represents hair being loosened — "letting one's hair down," relaxing.

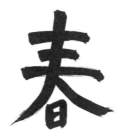

Chun - Spring season.
This character represents sun below and grass above, symbolizing spring has returned.

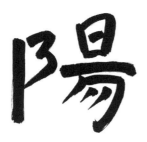

Yang - Positive principle in nature.
The left character is a mountain slope.
The top right side is the sun shining
on the slope and earth. Below the
horizontal line is a moon. This can
represent a body with the sun shining
on it or a worker bent over in the field
with sun on the back.

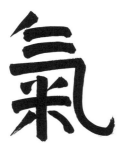

Qi (Chi) - Vital life force, energy.
Yang and qi together represent
positive intention or energy.

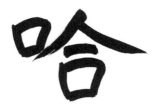

Ha - Laughter.
A mouth beside the character for
close or gather. This suggests the
opening and closing of the mouth
when laughing.

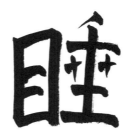

Shui - Sleep.
The left hand character represents
an eye. The right is the drooping
of the eye.

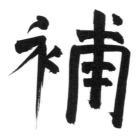

Bu - Nutrition, supply.
The character on the left is related
to clothing. The one on the right
has to do with food.

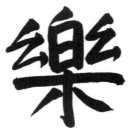

Le - Joy, happiness.
Also Yue - Music.
This character has silk strings surrounding a gong on top and below
the character for wood, which
could represent a music stand.
Music makes us joyful.

Balance

I am like a balance scale,
holding in my extended hands
the dualities that constitute my days.
The height of joy I sometimes reach
is measured by the depth I know.
A scale may fill one moment
and in the next tilt with the wind,
just as the day moves silently
to twilight, the dark to dawn.
Spring warmth may lift the scales
then let them fall beneath the weight of snow.

I must sink my roots deep into the soil of hope,
and hold steadfast in the winter's storm.
I shall place acceptance in one hand
and patience in the other
to find my equilibrium, that balm of equanimity I seek.

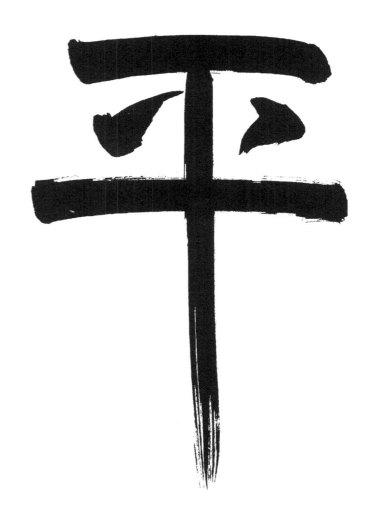

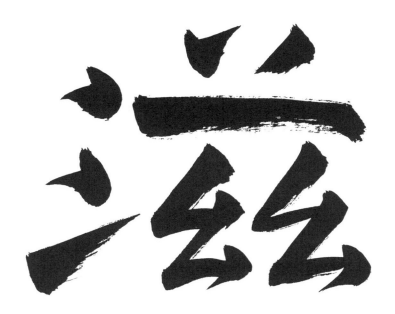

Nurture

I am the shepherd of my well being,

the shield that nurtures and befriends.

May I hold in my hands and in my heart,

the treasure of my life,

and cradle it in the shelter of my wing.

May my caring be an anchor:

the sentinel who sustains and succors,

that nourishes this road I travel.

May I be gentle with myself

and cherish who and what I am,

and may the mantle of this healing

fold gently down upon my shoulders.

Heart

Such a fragile thing this human heart

Its sheath so like the wings of butterflies;

Its dusting, once damaged, cannot catch the wind.

Let me cradle it always with a gentle hand

And cherish well each pulsing.

May I listen to its simple song.

Its bell-like melody speaks in a

Language far beyond the need for words

And asks that I bend low and bow my head

To hear the truth it softly sings.

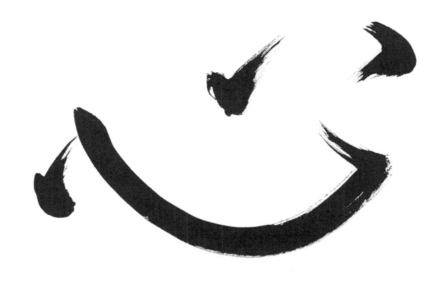

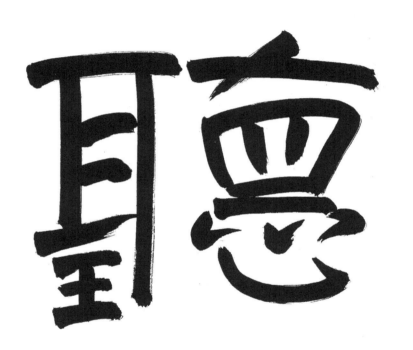

Listen

The labyrinth of my ear leads me
to the labyrinth of my touch,
for my fingers are antennas that listen to my world.

If I place them gently, devoid of any judgment,
they hear not only the beating of my heart
but the messages my body sings to me.

I listen best when my world is silent;
when the music of the body
whispers a melody I have known since my birth.

May I drink in these receptors of my soul.
May I hearken to the messages
my ears and fingers touch.
May my body be the shell I lift gently to my ear
so that I am wrapped in the messages my listening gives me.

Joy

Joy is the faithful healer of my soul,

a tuning fork that sings its canon

just beyond my hearing, just behind my ear.

It bubbles up like warm honey

from the middle of my belly

and melts its way into my hands

that reach for healing light.

It sparkles like a firefly in my darkness

and lifts my spirit in the night.

Its sweet music whispers in my ear,

a canticle in praise of hope.

It teaches me to dance.

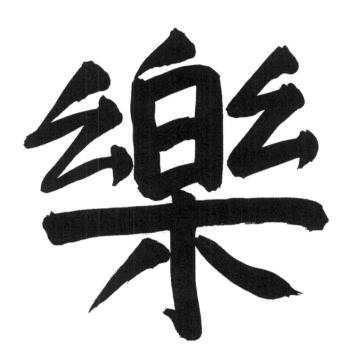

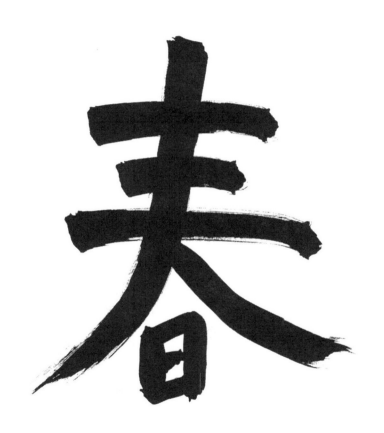

Spring

The pasture is a patchwork quilt

of snow and earth.

I dig my heel into the ground

to feel the give of soil.

Reluctant winter retreats

before the dancing hope of spring.

She skips in with promises

and I follow as she greens my world.

So gently does her mantle

drift down

upon the shoulders of the earth

to bring a singing

back into my winter heart.

I am tilting on her windmill into spring.

Resources

References

"Sometimes Healing Needs No Words" by Lois Bresee. Reprinted by permission of the author.

"Breathe" from *Call Me By My True Name* by Thich Nhat Hanh. Copyright ©1993 by Thich Nhat Hanh. Reprinted by permission of the author.

Haus, Diane, Illustrator. *Acupuncture Point Cards*. Jinan, China: Shandong Science and Technology Press, no date available. Reprinted by permission of the illustrator.

Konecne, Sharon, MHS, PT. "Treatment of Cancer Related Weakness and Fatigue." North American Seminars, course material, April 30 - May 1, 2005, Atlanta, GA.

Ladinsky, Daniel. "Laughter" from *I Heard God Laughing, Renderings of Hafiz*. Copyright © 2006 by Daniel Ladinsky. Reprinted by permission of Penguin Group Inc., New York.

Recommended Readings

Bauer, Cathryn. *Acupressure For Women*. Freedom, CA: The Crossing Press, 1987.

Cane, Pat, Ph.D. Living in Wellness: A *Capacitar CANCER Manual*. Capacitar International, www.capacitar.org.

Cane, Pat, Ph.D. *Trauma, Healing, & Transformation*. Capacitar International, www.capacitar.org.

Cargill, Marie. *Well Woman: Healing the Female Body through Traditional Chinese Medicine*. Westport, CT: Bergin & Garvey, 1998.

Chuen, Lam Wam. *The Way of Energy*. New York: Fireside Books, Simon & Schuster, 1991.

Dong, Y.P. *Still as a Mountain, Powerful as Thunder*. Boston, MA: Shambhala Publications, Inc., 1993.

Elias, Jason and Katherine Ketcham. *Chinese Medicine for Maximum Immunity*. New York: Three Rivers Press, 1998.

Elias, Jason and Katherine Ketcham. *In The House of the Moon: Reclaiming the Feminine Spirit of Healing*. New York: Warner Books Inc., 1995.

Gach, Michael Reed. *Acupressure's Potent Points: A Guide to Self-care for Common Ailments*. New York: Bantam Books, 1990.

Garropoli, Garri. *Qi Gong: Essence of the Healing Dance*. Deerfield Beach, FL: Health Communications, Inc., 1999.

Harpham, Wendy Schlessel. *After Cancer: A Guide to Your New Life*. New York: Harper Perennial, 1995.

Huang, Chungliang. *Embrace Tiger, Return to Mountain: The Essence of Tai Ji*. 3rd ed. Berkeley, CA: Celestial Arts, 1997.

Huang, Chungliang & Jerry Lynch. *Mentoring: The TAO of Giving and Receiving Wisdom*. San Francisco: Harper, 1995.

Johnson, Yanling Lee. *A Woman's Qigong Guide: Empowerment Through Movement, Diet and Herbs.* Boston: YMAA Publication Center, 2001.

Katzman, Shoshanna, L.Ac.,M.A. *Qigong For Staying Young.* New York: Avery, A Member of Penguin Group (USA) Inc., 2003.

Lewis, Dennis. *Free Your Breath, Free Your Life.* Boston, MA: Shambhala Publications, Inc., 2004.

Liang, Shou-Yu and Wen-Ching Wu. *Qigong Empowerment.* East Providence, RI: The Way of the Dragon Publishing, 1996.

Love, Dr. Susan. *Breast Book. 2nd ed.* Reading, MA: Perseus Books, 1995.

Nepo, Mark. *The Book of Awakening.* York Beach, ME: Conari Press, 2000.

Swirsky, Joan, R.N. and Diane Sackett Nannery. *Coping With Lymphedema.* New York: Avery Penguin Putnam, 1998.

Weiss, Maria C, M.D. and Ellen Weiss. *Living Beyond Breast Cancer: A Survivor's Guide for when Treatment Ends and the Rest of Your Life Begins.* New York: Times Books, 1998.

Additional Resources

Atlanta Lesbian Health Initiative, provides health education, focuses on the needs of the lesbian community. www.thehealthinitiative.org.

Cancer Lifeline, offers exercise programs for breast cancer survivors. Telephone: 800-255-5505 www.cancerlifeline.org.

CancerNet – National Institute of Health's information service on cancer-related topics. www.cancernet.nci.nih.gov.

CAPACITAR International, An International Project of Empowerment and Solidarity, teaches wellness practices, team building, and self-development. www.capacitar.org.

Celebrating Life Foundation, breast cancer awareness for women of color, local support groups, educational programs, other resources. 800-207-0992, www.celebratinglife.org.

Journey to Wellness, an on-line health magazine targeting ethnic minorities, provides health care and health literacy via the internet and radio programming. www.journeytowellness.com.

Living Beyond Breast Cancer, promotes health through workshops, newsletters, conferences, and telephone help line. 610-645-4567.

Mautner Project for Lesbians with Cancer, direct services, advocacy, and education. 202-332-5536, www.mautnerproject.org.

The National Lymphedema Network, excellent resource for lymphedema management. 510-208-3200, www.lymphnet.org.

Sisters...By Choice, Inc., a non-profit organization offering support through counseling, medical technology, education, and emotional support. www.sistersbychoice.net.

Sisters of Hope, support group for African-American women with breast cancer. 253-572-2683, sistersofhope@hotmail.com.

Susan G. Komen Breast Cancer Foundation. Telephone 877-GO-KOMEN www.komen.org.

Team Survivor, a program of the YWCA, offers exercise programs and other services for breast cancer survivors. Telephone 900-95-EPLUS, www.ywca.org.

The Wellness Community, emotional support, education, and hope. 888-783-WELL, www.thewellnesscommunity.org.

Contributors

Credits

Photos, Used with Permission

Yada Claassen: *pp. 25, 27, 28, 36, 37, 39, 40, 42, 43, 44, 58.*

William F. Hull: *pp. 29, 30, 31, 32, 33, 34, 35, 38, 41, 45.*

Calligraphy

Meg. Randolph

Illustrations

Diane Haus: *pp. 47, 48, 49, 50, 51, 52, 53, 54.*

Meg. Randolph: *p. 57.*

Cielle Tewksbury: *pp. 19, 21, 56.*

Anecdotes

Meredith Morgan: *p. 10*

Sally Peavy: *p. 9*

Layout & Design

Lucy Hohn

Text Editing

Leslie Richardson

Mary Brown Sinclair

Acknowledgments

CAPACITAR International

Janet Goodridge

Jo & Jim McLean

Chungliang Huang

Sally Yu Liang Huang

Pearl Weng Liang Huang

Alex Chao Liang Huang

Polly Sundari Maliongas

John & Pat Randolph

Susan E. Robertson

About the Authors

Meg. Randolph, MS, PT, has practiced physical therapy since 1977. She began her Tai Ji and Qi Gong practice in 1994. She is currently a Tai Ji student of Chungliang Huang of the Living Tao Foundation and has also studied with Wei Lun Huang, Cielle Tewksbury, Dr. Paul Lam, and Diirga Brough. Meg. continues her physical therapy practice, focusing on a blend of Eastern and Western techniques and is committed to serving people whose access to health care is limited.

In addition to working in acute hospital care, Meg. has worked in community health and wellness since the early 1970s. She is certified by Dr. Paul Lam to teach Tai Chi for Arthritis and Tai Chi for Back Pain. She teaches Tai Ji and Qi Gong in Atlanta and offers workshops throughout the southeastern United States and in Central America.

Cielle Tewksbury received her BA degree in liberal arts from Norwich University with a concentration in Cross Cultural Dance Anthropology and Comparative Religion. She received her dance training from the American School of Dance and the Bella Lewitsky Dance Company.

For the past 20 years, Cielle has been a Senior Instructor with Tai Ji Master, Chungliang Al Huang of the Living Tao Foundation. Lawrence Galante and Paul Gallagher were her instructors in Yang style Tai Chi Chuan. She offers seminars in Tai Ji, Qi Gong, Mudras, Chinese sabre and fan to participants across the United States and in Europe. She is a certified Labyrinth Facilitator with Grace Cathedral in San Francisco and has spent three summers at Chartres Cathedral in France as part of their annual labyrinth program.

Meg. Randolph and Cielle Tewksbury are available for Qi Gong workshops in Hospital Cancer Centers throughout the U.S., Europe, and Latin America. To contact us: e-mail healinggiftsqigong@gmail.com.